V. A. BOMA

10 QUESTIONS EVERYONE SHOULD ASK THEIR PHARMACIST

DEADLY MISTAKES PATIENTS OVERLOOK

Ⓟ
PHARMACY-MEDICATION SMART
Know your medicine

This book was professionally typeset on Reedsy.
Find out more at reedsy.com

This book is dedicated to all the pharmacists that work everyday to prevent medication errors, and to all the families that have experienced some form of medication error.

Contents

Table of Contents

10 Questions Everyone Should Their Pharmacist
Deadly mistakes Patients overlook
Quick Reference Guide

- **Introduction**
- **Statistics**
- **The Practice of Pharmacy Today**

Ten Questions to Ask Your Pharmacist

1. Have you verified my name and Date of birth?
2. What is the name of my medication?
3. What is my medication indicated (use) for?
4. Have you verified my drug allergies?
5. Can I take this medication if I am pregnant?
6. Are there any food-Drug interactions?
7. Are there any Drug -Drug interactions?
8. Do I need to do blood work when I take this medication?
9. How long should I be on this medication?9
10. Can I take my prescription with me on vacation longer than a month?

- **<u>Bonus Question:</u> Can I drive a car or operate machinery while taking this medication?**
- **Conclusion**

Introduction

After more than *20 years* in the pharmaceutical and healthcare system, I felt that it's my duty to reach out to anyone who has ever had a question about a medication they are taking and just never felt like they were listened to, or that their questions and concerns were never properly addressed. If you can relate to this, then this book is intended for **you**.

My dear reader, thanks for picking up this book to read. I am assuming either you or a family member is taking medication today to treat an ailment. This includes over the counter medications, which do not require a prescription and can still impact your life in a positive or negative way if taken incorrectly. Hopefully, you find this information useful, and if you do, please educate, and share with your family, friends, and loved ones.

This quick reference guide is a simplified, made-easy-to-read book to help the reader understand the basics when it comes to medication errors and safety. The title "10 Questions That Everyone Should Ask Their Pharmacist" was created and intended to prevent medication mishaps. If you are a patient or have loved ones receiving any kind of medications, like prescriptions from their doctor's office or just buying an over-the-counter medication from their major retail shops, this book will be a useful tool to have. When you are armed with this set of 10 questions and answers, the probability that you will be a victim of medication errors is very slim. This is not an all-inclusive book, but the next version will dive more into other aspects of medication errors and adverse drug events that are killing millions of people around the world today. It only takes one of the 10 questions listed not properly implemented to cause serious harm to a patient, including death. Therefore, I recommend you read and share this book with all your loved ones, especially your elderly family members, parents of children, and most importantly pediatric or young infants. The listed group has a higher risk of intolerance to medications. As we age, our organ functions will decline, and our kidneys will not be as effective as they were when we were young adults. Thus, medication clearance is less, and this can lead to toxicity. With the pediatric population, their organs are not fully developed, so their medications must be calculated based on different parameters like their height, age, weight, etc. to avoid any adverse events or medication errors. Some insurance companies are willing to hire pharmacists to attend medical rounds in hospitals and make recommendations to physicians regarding patient medication needs. Unfortunately, this is less common in retail settings. It is vital to have a pharmacist available while a medication is being prescribed on a medical team while a medication is being prescribed. Several studies have shown that the presence of a pharmacist on a medical team reduces the occurrence of medication errors. This is important as to prevent common medication errors, especially in institutions where new resident physicians are still undergoing their residency training. Unfortunately, in outpatient physician offices, this service is not available, so any error made while prescribing may not be caught by their outpatient setting pharmacist. This can be fatal combined with the busy schedule of most outpatient pharmacists, as I will discuss in the next chapter because this topic warrants more discussion on how such incidents should be mitigated. Hopefully the list of 10 questions will be the rule of practice on a daily basis, even if the pharmacist is busy. You can all attest that in large retail pharmacies, it's practically impossible to talk with a pharmacist, and that should be the patient's first point of contact. Unfortunately, that is not the case except if the patient is receiving a new medication or prescription, which is a requirement warranted by some pharmacy state board organizations. What happens if that new medication may interact with a new over the counter medication or other prescriptions?

This book is for informational purposes only and should not override the decisions of your personal physician and pharmacist

Statistics

The U.S. Census Bureau QuickFacts: United States (2021) states that the US Population as of July 1st, 2021, is estimated to be about 331,893,745. According to the article "Prescription Drugs" (2019),"more than 131 million people take prescription drugs, and this is especially higher in the elderly population and patients with chronic conditions". According to the organization Partnership to End Addiction (2013), "Almost 70 percent of Americans take at least one prescription medication, and more than half take at least two, according to a new study by researchers at the Mayo Clinic". With this high level of drug utilization, close monitoring is essential to avoid medication errors that can lead to death. Also, The Center for Drug Evaluation and Research (2019) defines a medication error as "any preventable event that may cause or lead to inappropriate medication use or patient harm while the medication is in the control of the healthcare professional, patient, or consumer". Unfortunately, medication errors are happening every day. In the article "Study Suggests Medical Errors Now Third Leading Cause of Death in the US" (2016), "more than 250,000 people in the U.S. die every year from medical errors". And medical errors are the third-leading cause of death after heart disease and cancer. With respect to medical errors, according to research by da Silva and Krishnamurthy (2016), "medication errors harm an estimated 1.5 million people every year, costing at least $3.5 billion annually. It is estimated that ADEs [Adverse Drug Events] affect approximately 2 million hospital stays annually and prolong the length of stay by 1.7–4.6 days".

Based on the statistical data I just referenced it is obvious why we need to place a lot of emphasis on patient safety and to create a system in place to mitigate such occurrences. I truly believe most of these errors are avoidable is at most ten of the questions and answers are listed below are implemented as a standard of care or procedures to be followed before any medication is dispense or administered to a patient. Hopefully by reading this article you will gain some insights on how to navigate our robust and sometimes very complicated medical system. Thus, help reduce medication mishaps from affecting your loved ones.

The Practice of Pharmacy Today

I n the early 1900s, pharmacists acted as apothecaries and they compounded medications. This led to them spending a lot of time understanding their patients' medications and helped them create an intimate relationship with their patients. As the years went by, the 1950 pharmaceutical companies took the role of manufacturing prescriptions, and this impacted the role of pharmacist. Initially, this was seen as a positive move to take the pharmacist away from compounding to focusing on patient care. Unfortunately, this has been very difficult to accomplish, especially in retail settings.

Pharmacists are required to spend 7 years gaining in depth knowledge about the role of medication and its impact if taken correctly or incorrectly. In 2000 it was a requirement for Pharmacists to Have a Doctorate (PharmD) to be licensed to practice pharmacy. Unfortunately, that knowledge is not properly utilized because of the setting they are required to work in, especially in retail pharmacy settings where the number of prescriptions you dispense has overshadowed patient safety. So, for pharmacists to keep their jobs, they unintentionally are spending less time reviewing and verifying their patient's prescription, which has led to the errors we described above. After thorough consideration and my passion for patient safety, I decided to write down at least 10 questions every patient should ask their pharmacist when they pick up their medication. These questions will help save the lives of our family members and loved one.

Question 1: Have You Verified My Name and Date of Birth?

This is a question that should always be asked because in the pharmacy system, we can have fifty patients and more with the same last name. The best way to avoid dispensing the wrong medication to the wrong patient is to always make sure they repeat your date of birth or at least your month and year of birth. A lot of errors have occurred because the wrong patient was given someone else's medication because of their similar names. Can you imagine how many patients have the same first and last names? So if emphasis is not placed on their date of birth, this can lead to unforeseen and sometimes deadly consequences. Please always ask your pharmacist your date of birth or at least your month and day of birth if privacy is warranted.

Question 2: What is the Name of My Medication?

This should always be asked because there is a common term in pharmacy called SALADs (Sound-Alike Look-Alike Drugs), referring to look-alike and sound-alike drug names and look-alike product packaging, which can cause confusion resulting in potentially harmful medication errors. There have been several instances where patients have received a completely different medication from what was prescribed because of the name and sometimes pill size and color similarities. A typical example could be a patient who has never had diabetes that was given an oral diabetes medication because the medications sounded like one another. An example of this could be Chlorpromazine used for nausea and Chlorpropamide used to lower blood sugar levels or diabetes, where these medications end up being switched with each other. Another example is a patient who has never had high blood pressure who was given medication for that indication. Such errors can lead to fatalities. Another example could be a patient who has allergies that was given an antidepressant. An example of this could be Cetirizine that is used for allergies and Sertraline that is used for depression being switched with each other. Another example may include Clonidine that is used for blood pressure and Clonazepam that is used for anxiety being switched with each other. The last example that I will include here is Cyclosporine that is used for transplant patients being switched with Cycloserine used for Tuberculosis. This is not an all-inclusive list. Unfortunately, these types of errors occur every day and have led to coma and death in some patients. A non-diabetic patient being given a diabetic medication will lead to severe hypoglycemia, coma, and sometimes death. These are fatalities that can be avoided if you verify the name of your medication with the pharmacist every time you pick it up from the store. Unfortunately, in retail pharmacy settings where the pharmacy is the last point of contact for the patient, once the types of errors listed above happen it can lead to deadly consequences. At least in the hospital setting where the nurse is the last point of contact for the patient, this might provide another cushion of safety because the nurse is required to verify the medication before administering. Regardless, even with this line of defense, we still have medication errors in hospital settings as well.

Question 3: What is My Medication Indicated (Used) For?

You always must ask your pharmacist what your medication is indicated or used for because one medication can have several indications or uses. Sometimes the strength or dose of a medication is what determines its indication. A typical example is 150mg of Bupropion being used for smoking cessation, while the other doses of bupropion are used for depressive disorder. Another example is 20mg of Tadalafil being used to treat Pulmonary Arterial Hypertension (PAH), 5mg of Tadalafil being used to treat Benign Prostatic Hypertrophy (BPH), and other doses of Tadalafil being used for erectile dysfunction. By asking this question, the pharmacist is obliged to review your medication profile to make sure you have the disease that this medication is indicated for. There have been instances where an error was prevented because while reviewing the patient's profile, the pharmacist realized that medication was for another patient. This alone can cause severe harm, leading to death. Patients have been in a coma because they were given medication to treat diabetes or hypertension, and they were neither hypertensive or diabetic. Always ask.

Question 4: Have You Verified My Drug Allergies?

Drug allergies are another leading cause of mishap when not documented properly for the pharmacist to review before dispensing a medication. We've had instances where patients were allergic to penicillin, completely ignored or never documented in the pharmacy system, and this resulted in severe anaphylactic reactions. So, always verify if your drug allergy information is documented in the system. Other instances might concern the actual drug you are allergic to, but we have what is called "cross sensitivity". Implying that if you are allergic to one class of drugs, you are likely to also be allergic to another class of drugs. This usually happens because these drugs share a similar chemical structure, even though sometimes they belong to a completely different class. A typical example may involve a patient that has a penicillin allergy who may be allergic to Cephalosporin. A patient that develops angioedema on an Angiotensin Blocking Agent (ACE) inhibitor used for blood pressure may be allergic to an Angiotensin Receptor Antagonist (ARB) also used for blood pressure. This is just to list a few, and that is why it is vital to tell your pharmacist all your drug allergies and food allergies.

Question 5: Can I Take This Medication if I am Pregnant?

Another mishap that can occur is taking medication that can be dangerous for your fetus. You should always ask your pharmacist if you can take a certain medication prescribed, especially if you are in the child-bearing age and not taking any family planning precautions. This serious question can avoid birth defects like cleft palates. Medications are usually classified by pregnancy categories. So, a medication is safer if it belongs to a pregnancy Category B, but sometimes a certain medication may be prescribed that falls into pregnancy Category C, etc. It is always recommended to verify with your pharmacist if your medication is safe in the chance that you are pregnant or plan to get pregnant. As you can imagine, some women of child-bearing age are required and freeze their eggs before chemotherapy. When we talk of women in the child-bearing age, we forget about men partnered up with these same women of child-bearing age. Why is this important? Well, there are medications that if consumed by your spouse, you may have to avoid sexual intercourse for some time. This is because of the medication(s) potential effects on the fetus. Men are also affected by medications that can reduce their sperm count and sometimes result in erectile dysfunction. So please, always ask your pharmacist about the safety of your medications if you plan to have a family.

Question 6: Are There Any Drug-Food Interactions?

D rug-food interaction is another important question to ask your pharmacist about. A typical example includes blood thinners like Warfarin. While on blood thinners, patients should avoid other medications or foods high in vitamin K to prevent them from bleeding to death. Another drug-food interaction that people tend to ignore is alcohol. Taking your medications and drinking alcohol can be very fatal, especially when combined with the drug family of Benzodiazepines, primarily used for anxiety. This Benzodiazepine family includes medications like Clonazepam and Alprazolam. Opioids and opioid-derivatives like Codeine and Methadone also tend to be mixed a lot with alcohol. Consuming alcohol with the former can lead to severe drowsiness. Consuming alcohol with opioids can lead to respiratory depression. Some patients take Methadone, an opioid-derivative used for drug addiction or pain, and consume alcohol at the same time, while also mixing them with Benzodiazepine mentioned above. This has killed a lot of famous and not-so-famous people, so no one is immune from this deadly combination of medications. We have seen on TV instances where someone went to bed and never woke up because of the deadly effects of taking Methadone with alcohol or Benzodiazepine. Please, use caution and always ask your pharmacist what medications or foods should be completely avoided when on certain medications. If not, this can lead to severe unpleasant side effects, and sometimes medications might be less effective like antibiotics when combined with alcohol. Also, some medications are required to be taken on an empty stomach to be effective. Therefore, asking this question is very important mitigate the risk of not getting the beneficial effect from your medication.

Question 7: Are There Any Drug-Drug Interactions?

D rug-drug interaction is one of the most common medication errors, especially with patients taking sometimes ten medications and more. You can still have drug-drug interaction with just two medications. Patients practicing polypharmacy are at a greater risk of having drug-drug interaction medication errors. This is avoidable by asking your pharmacist if they have reviewed your medication profile or medication list to make sure there are no drug-drug interactions or contraindications. Remember to tell your pharmacist what other medications you are taking over the counter. If you fill your prescriptions at different pharmacies, which should be greatly discouraged, always ask your pharmacist to give you your most recent medication list. Make sure you give them a medication list from your other pharmacies so that a comprehensive list can be created in their system. This will help prevent drug-drug interaction related errors which can be very fatal.

Question 8: Do I Need to do Blood work When I Take This Medication?

To be able to take certain medications and to also avoid drug toxicity, blood work will be required. Your pharmacist should be able to tell you which medications on your profile require blood work. Your physician should have also probably mentioned this to you as well. To avoid mishap and even death, blood work is very important for certain medications like Warfarin, which is a blood thinner. There are many other medications not mentioned. This will be elaborated on future write ups.

Question 9: How Long Should I be on This Medication?

S ome medications are required to be taken for life, and some medications are indicated only to be taken for a few days. Certain medications for allergies, which are seasonal, are indicated to be taken usually around spring when the pollen counts are very high, and most antibiotics are usually for short-term therapy. Sometimes prolonged consumption of antibiotics can be detrimental to your health, along with some over the counter medications where there is hardly any stop-dates on their labels. Prolonged use of antibiotics beyond the prescribed stop date can destroy your normal flora or your gut bacteria needed to protect your gut. It's always advised to ask your pharmacist how long you should be taking your medications or the duration of time your medicine has been prescribed to be taken to avoid some of the consequences I just listed above.

Question 10: Can I Take My Prescription With Me on Vacation Longer Than a Month?

I have seen cases where patients are not able to verify what they will need from the pharmacist if they must travel for more than a month. This is a very important question to ask. Many cases involve patients avoiding asking for help due to their insurance plan carrier. If you plan to stay for travel within the United States and have access to one of the large chain pharmacies, you can always transfer your prescription to another pharmacy when you get to your destination. You will have to take your prescription information to the pharmacy of your choice and ask the pharmacist to initiate a transfer of your prescription to them. This must be done by the transferring pharmacy. Give the pharmacy the information of your old pharmacy, and they will call them. Another situation may be if you are traveling out of the United States and you need more than a 30-day supply, but your insurance plan only provides a maximum of a 30-day supply. My recommendation is for you to call your insurance prescription plan and let them know your plan. They should likely approve more than a 30-day supply. Another option is to call your pharmacist to initiate and facilitate this process. Leaving for vacation without enough medications is unsafe, especially for patients with chronic conditions like diabetes, asthma, hypertension, seizures, and some psychiatric disorders just to list a few. Abruptly stopping your medication can lead to severe withdrawal effects and even rebound hypertension on certain anti hypertensive medications like Clonidine, and severe anxiety can come about after stopping Clonazepam or Sertraline. The insurance company may be willing to give you a supply that is enough to the extent that you can justify that you will be gone for a while. So please, always ask your pharmacist to help you get some extra days of your medications when traveling.

Bonus Question: Can I Drive a Car or Operate Machinery While Taking This Medication?

The answer is yes and no depending on the medication. Some medications you can take while driving and operating machinery and some medications you cannot. The next book will discuss this and other desirable topics in depth. Hope you enjoyed the short read, and please make sure you share with all your family members and friends to avoid these common fatal and sometimes deathly medication mishaps.

Conclusion

After working and spending more than 20 years in the medical profession, I have seen so many avoidable occurrences. I have always felt that it's my duty to reach out to educate and tell people what to do to avoid such occurrences. I am hoping that what I wrote will help someone who has unanswered questions or who needs help navigating our pharmaceutical or medication-dispensing system. I decided to make this very short to allow those who just want to know what questions to ask their pharmacist before they take any medications home to navigate through this book quickly. This is a very sensitive and personal issue, and many families have been traumatized because of lack of accessibility to their pharmacist. Pharmacists went to school to provide the services I just listed, and unfortunately their working environments do not give them the ability to practice as it was intended. The number of scripts or prescriptions they can fill a day determine their job security, and by doing so, patients, family members, and loved ones are at risk of becoming victims of the most common medical errors harming at least 1.5 million people every year. I do look forward to writing on more relatable topics and will love your feedback. Thanks for reading as always.

References

Center for Drug Evaluation and Research. (2019, August 23). *Working to Reduce Medication Errors.* U.S. Food and Drug Administration. https://www.fda.gov/drugs/information-consumers-and-patients-drugs/work

Ing-reduce-medication-errors

da Silva, B., MD, & Krishnamurthy, M., MD, FACP, SFHM. (2016, September 7).
The alarming reality of medication error: a patient case and review of Pennsylvania and National data. National Library of Medicine. https://www.ncbi.nlm.nih.gov/pmc/articles/PMC5016741/#:%7E:text=Medic

ation%20errors%20harm%20an%20estimated, (3) %20(N).

NCBI - WWW Error Blocked Diagnostic. (2016, September 7). National Library of
Medicine.
https://www.ncbi.nlm.nih.gov/pmc/articles/PMC5016741/#:%7E:text=Medic

ation%20errors%20harm%20an%20estimated, (3)%20(N).

Partnership to End Addiction. (2013, June 20). *Almost 70 Percent of Americans*
  Take at Least One Prescription Medication, Study Finds.
  https://drugfree.org/drug-and-alcohol-news/almost-70-percent-of-american
  s-take-at-least-one-prescription-medication-study-finds/

Prescription Drugs. (2019, February 13). Health Policy Institute.
  https://hpi.georgetown.edu/rxdrugs/

Study Suggests Medical Errors Now Third Leading Cause of Death in the U.S.
  (2016, May 3). Hopkins Medicine.
  https://www.hopkinsmedicine.org/news/media/releases/study_su
  ggests_m
  edical_errors_now_third_leading_cause_of_death_in_the_us

U.S. Census Bureau QuickFacts: United States. (2021, July 1). Census Bureau
  QuickFacts. https://www.census.gov/quickfacts/fact/table/US/PS
  T045221

Printed in Great Britain
by Amazon